In God's Hands

In God's Hands

Living Through Illness with Faith

Maureen A. Cummings

Our Sunday Visitor

www.osv.com
Our Sunday Visitor Publishing Division
Our Sunday Visitor, Inc.
Huntington, Indiana 46750

Copyright © 2018 by Maureen A. Cummings. Published 2018.

23 22 21 20 19 18   1 2 3 4 5 6 7 8 9

Our Sunday Visitor Publishing Division
Our Sunday Visitor, Inc.
200 Noll Plaza
Huntington, IN 46750
1-800-348-2440

ISBN: 978-1-68192-185-3 (Inventory No. T1894)
eISBN: 978-1-68192-189-1
LCCN: 2018935817

Cover and interior design: Amanda Falk
Cover art: Shutterstock
Interior art: Photo of Maureen A. Cummings courtesy of the author.

PRINTED IN THE UNITED STATES OF AMERICA

About the Author

Maureen Cummings is a cradle Catholic, wife and mother of six, and a Secular Franciscan. A homeschooling parent for over 25 years, she now writes from Janesville, Wisconsin. *In God's Hands* is Maureen's first book.

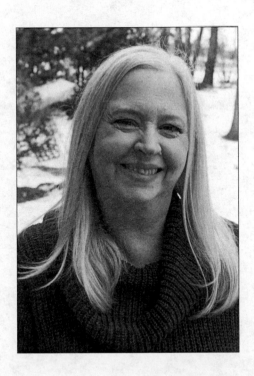

*To all those who suffer
and to those who help
them in their time of need.*

"My destiny is in your hands;
rescue me from my enemies,
from the hands of my pursuers."
— PSALM 31:16

Upon receiving news of a serious medical diagnosis, you
may feel alone, you may feel overwhelmed, you may feel
hopeless. I know I did. But I believe that with God's help,
whether you are a patient, a friend, or a family member, you
will find strength and peace in God's hands.

TABLE OF CONTENTS

Chapter One

WHY NOT ME?

For I know well the plans I have in mind for you —
oracle of the LORD — plans for your welfare and
not for woe, so as to give you a future of hope.
— JEREMIAH 29:11

February in the Midwest is invariably cold and gray. Snow can be a pretty blessing (and sometimes a curse), but it also turns gray and tarnished. It is too far from Christmas and too long until spring. I have often been glad that it has the fewest days of any month.

In the midst of a cold and dreary February day, when I thought I had discovered a breast infection, it was just one more thing. I was still nursing my sixth child and had never had an infection, so I just figured it was my turn. After a few days, I went to the doctor, whom I knew well, and joked that at least it was not cancer. The joke was on me. I was forty-two years old, with an eight-month-old nursing baby plus five other children, when I was told that I had stage III breast cancer.

Just Breathe

The shock of a major medical diagnosis is one that many, if not most of us, will someday face. It affects not only the patients but also all those around them, from friends and family to neighbors and coworkers. No matter what the diagnosis — cancer, heart disease, diabetes, Alzheimer's, or kidney failure — it always comes as a shock. Even if the warning signs are there — family history, obesity, smoking, whatever — a major illness is always as unexpected as it is unwelcome.

First aid courses teach us to respond to shock with warmth, rest, and a patient watchfulness. Sounds great. But the medical professionals who teach us those simple steps throw most of that out the window and replace it with a cra-

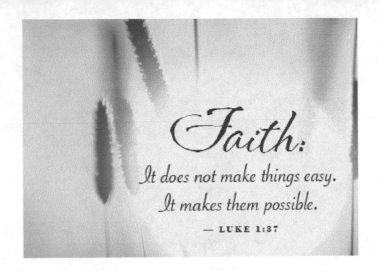

Faith:

It does not make things easy.
It makes them possible.

— LUKE 1:37

January, 2020

Dear family,

We were looking for something that we felt would support Pat and Joan too, and we ran across this book, "In God's Hands". After reading it, we felt the words and experiences in it would bring us all strength in our time of need whether we were the one with the illness or the care giver for a loved one. We hope y'all will find encouragement and hope as we did.

Our love and God bless,

Tim & Elaine

Tim & Elaine

zy train of appointments, labs, tests, counselors, and therapies. This is their job, and they are good at it.

So, you or someone you love has received a serious diagnosis? Please, literally, take a breath. Whatever thoughts are running around your brain, take them to God. It is not necessary to go to a church or anywhere else. Just ask God to help you process this news. It takes some sorting and letting go as emotions swing from shock to anger to relief at knowing that what has been wrong for months was not in your imagination. Fear is there, too, and it will pop up on a regular basis.

Perhaps some of you reading this can handle your diagnosis, and all it will entail, hand it over to God, and be at peace with whatever happens. That would be wonderful. Truly. I was blessed in that I could give my new situation to God — for about thirty seconds. Then I took all the problems back, told him what I thought should happen (and should not have happened), demanded to know what was going on, begged to see my children grow up, ranted about whatever I was currently thinking about, and then started the cycle again. I am not proud of this, but it is true. Some of you may be so angry with God that you do not even want to talk to him about anything. Others are ready to accept what is happening, but their loved ones are not.

You Don't Have to Do It Alone

If possible, stop by a church or other place of prayer and just sit. Do nothing. Let God give you first aid. It may seem silly and futile to sit in an empty church. But go, if at all possible. And if you are Catholic (or even if you're not), try to find time for Eucharistic Adoration. This is a time when the Holy Eucharist is present on the altar and made visible in a beautiful vessel called a monstrance. Some parishes do not have a regular time for Adoration, while others may have a chapel with twenty-four-hour Adoration. The point is to find a holy, quiet spot. Let God — who, after all, gave you your life — help your brain sort through all the information and feelings that have flooded into and over you after this diagnosis. Loved ones, too, are shocked and in need of his care. Will some miracle take place? Probably not in the normal sense. But at this early stage, just getting some room to breathe is a miracle you will appreciate. Wherever you are, even in the doctor's office, ask God for graces. Ask for the grace you know you need, and then ask him to throw in whatever else he's got — which is a lot. Then remind yourself to be open to that grace.

One of the first graces I received was three simple words: "Why not me?" With no history of breast cancer in parents, grandparents, or siblings, it seemed odd at best. With having breastfed five children, and doing so with the sixth child at the time (it is very rare to be diagnosed with breast cancer while nursing), I was prepared for a "why me" refrain in my head. But what I heard was a little, tiny voice saying, "Why *not* me?" I am just as selfish and fearful of my own mortality as the average Joe, so I knew this was not *my* thought but someone else's. True, I "should" not have gotten cancer. I did not want cancer. But there it was.

Why *not* me?

Emotional Rollercoaster

This rollercoaster of feelings and emotions often continues for both the patient and those around the patient throughout — and even after — treatment. You may even switch places and positions. For example, at the beginning of this journey, a family member or caregiver may have a positive, take-charge attitude, while the patient is in total denial that anything is wrong. Weeks later, the family member or caregiver may not accept the changes the diagnosis is going to entail in life, while the patient is ready to charge ahead. It is not a matter of miscommunication. Rather, it is just two humans struggling with the same situation but from different perspectives. These changes can result in confusion, or even anger.

Just like on a rollercoaster one goes from screaming to laughter, it is best to realize that both caretaker and patient are in for a heck of a ride. If you can find the strength and the faith to invite God along, the twists and turns can sometimes even bring unexpected joy and laughter. The Catholic Church offers tons of help, whether you have practiced your faith all along or not. If you have wandered away over the years, now is a great time to return. No matter what the diagnosis, and no matter how your story unfolds, God is your best buddy on the rollercoaster ride of your life.

Find Support

With any medical situation, there can be bad outcomes. Isn't that a nice way of putting it? No one says that when you are getting into the car to get groceries, but there can be bad outcomes there too. Anyway, there are some things you can prepare for in advance. Surprising to me were the adults who felt the need to share their own fears. My first, and unkind, response was to be really ticked off with these people. Why would anyone call a newly diagnosed person to tell them horror stories of a great aunt who died painfully, or of a father who wasted away before their eyes of the same disease or condition? I was raised to be polite, so I was polite — until I got off the phone. Then I would rant and rave to any adult I could find about how people were crazy!

For some reason, I kept getting this type of call. Do not be surprised if you get them as well. I kept being superficially polite until God helped me realize that these callers were more scared than I was; that they had lived with these fears — fears that were new to me — for years. Although I'm sure they didn't realize it, these conversations were a call for help with their own fears. The lesson for me was to stop being selfish, to really listen, and to try to console them. It should not make any difference that I was scared too: *they* needed help, and I could give it — just by listening.

Listen

So, besides learning about my disease and everything that went with it, I began to understand that my new job was to listen. This change in attitude had three effects. First, it reminded me of how fragile and lonely we humans can be. This is humbling. Second, it encouraged me to think about and pray for others. Praying for others is always a good thing. Third, it made me realize that focusing on myself during this time would, at least for me, not be a good thing.

The fragility of those who called me reminded me of my own fears, but also of how we all have these fears.

Listening to others' sad memories and worries about their own futures helped me to face my own. It also helped me to thank God for all the things others had faced, but I had not. I could not do much for them; just tell them how treatments had changed dramatically, and how they were kind to think of me. I would ask for their prayers and mean it, knowing they would do so in whatever way they could. Eventually — though it took a while — I even felt joy that I could help them a tiny bit, all the while they were trying in their own way to help me. Just as I was finding joy in the phone calls, they dried up. God had gotten my attention, led me to think of others, and poof! That was it. It was back down the rollercoaster — focusing and worrying about myself with the newly added realization that selfish self-awareness was not a good choice.

Giving Help

Even if we don't feel like helping, we usually do it because we know we will feel better when we do, and perhaps guilty if we don't. It makes us look good too. Helping can even be fun. My parents set a wonderful example of helping others, so I grew up knowing how to help. I just had never been on the other side.

I did not know how to receive help, and I did not really want to know. Whether ignorantly or cold-heartedly, I had never thought much about the person on the other end of that assistance — except that they got frosting on their cake, and we were lucky to get powdered sugar sprinkled on ours.

If you are a friend, you can give aid and then go back to your normal life. If you are a caregiver, you can "help" and then, maybe, walk away or at least run errands. This is not true for the person who is on the receiving end of that aid. Hopefully, we are grateful for the help we receive. But we are also still stuck with the new situation that makes receiving help suddenly part of our lives.

Accepting Help

Independence and self-reliance are in the American bloodstream. It is true for both men and women. Whether it is cowboy movies or superheroes, we grow up believing that we are supposed to be the strong, take-charge heroes of life; that we should save others and rely on no one, except maybe in the final scenes for a happy story wrap-up. The thing is that with any major disease, at some point you are going to need help. I did not want to "need" help. Maybe you do not want to "need" help (or be a burden to anyone else) either.

It took me quite some time, and a few moments of resentment, to figure out that I was not just a recipient of aid but rather part of a wonderful movement of grace. If I could thankfully receive help from others, I was actually part of an exchange of grace and blessings. This new circumstance of having a major illness forced me to accept help. That was inevitable. *How* I accepted it? That was within my control.

People need to help each other on a deep level. Christians who learn the spiritual and corporal works of mercy know that it is just part of who we are as individual believers and as a Church. Being sick can lead us to being a blessing to others. Our illness also allows others to be a blessing to us. We should not deny them that opportunity for grace!

Be Not Afraid

The most difficult part of the serious illness journey is the temptation to give in to fear. The Bible says "Be not afraid" many, many times. Your faith, even if it is fragile or unsure, can make the difference for you on this rollercoaster. It will help you find peace and balance when there are challenges. At first, just pray — however, wherever, you can. Pray.

Odds are, you and your loved ones have been doing that interiorly ever since the medical diagnosis. Making it clear to yourself and to God that you are asking for his help, though, will give you a few moments of peace. Give it all to God — throw it at him if you need to (respectfully, if you can). He will not be upset if you are upset; he will just be glad you came to him. There may be times you have only him. He really can give you a sense of balance and peace in the midst of the craziness of a diagnosis. And moreover, he *wants* to.

Prayer does not need memorization, formulas, or books. You may want to close your eyes, grasp a rosary, get on your knees, or lift your head high. It is up to you. Talk to God, even if you haven't said much of anything to him in years. Tell him all that is on your heart. Then, straighten up, take a deep breath, and tell yourself to not be afraid — even if you are terrified. Like I was.

Chapter Two

LOOK FOR THE GOOD

I will praise you, LORD, with all my heart;
I will declare all your wondrous deeds.
— PSALM 9:2

You may have had your doubts, but you have survived at least the initial shock of your diagnosis. No matter what you're facing, though, there will continue to be challenging "aftershocks" and new things to learn about. Consider it a new school or a new unit study — one you probably didn't intend to sign up for! You will need to learn the vocabulary, procedures, purposes, and potential outcomes. There will be side journeys, new people in your life, and new places. There will be choices to make. Somewhere between recognizing your diagnosis and accepting it, there is a space where God can enter and help you tremendously. Here are six tools that make a difference.

Travel Light

Considering that this is not an unexpected, all-expenses-paid trip to Hawaii or Europe or Australia, it may be hard to imagine it as a journey of any sort — but it is. Any new journey offers an opportunity for a fresh start. You make a new packing list. You set aside clean clothes. You keep necessary new purchases in a special place. You may even clean your house or apartment so that it is neat and tidy when you return. In addition, it is usually best to travel as lightly as possible. The less and lighter the luggage, the easier it is to travel through an airport, by a ship, or even just to a hotel. Traveling light also leaves room to pick up souvenirs and gifts that help you remember the good things that happen along the road.

So, before you start *this* new journey, consider making a fresh start and traveling light. You can begin by turning to the Lord to ask for forgiveness. If you are Catholic, this means going to the Sacrament of Penance and Reconciliation. Don't close the book! Remember: "Be not afraid!" Confession is a great gift. It is *not* preparation for the end. But it can be preparation for the journey you'll be taking, courtesy of a serious medical diagnosis. Confession lightens your load by taking away all your sins, and it gives you the grace you need for a fresh start. It is free, doesn't take much time, and it will recharge your spiritual life.

This is even more important if you have been away from the Church. On the practical side, if it has been years since your last confession, there are options other than just showing up at the scheduled times. It's possible to call and make an appointment. You can consult the websites of nearby parishes to see when confession is offered. No one will even know. Maybe just write down the phone number, or ask someone you know to pick up a bulletin from a local church. If you do decide to go, don't worry: no one is going to yell at you. Every priest I know is thrilled whenever someone comes back to the church. If you cannot bring yourself to go to confession right now, just keep thinking and praying about it. Sooner is better, but our good God understands when we need to take baby steps.

Find a Focus

You will find that there is always more to learn about the illness that is affecting your life. When I was diagnosed with cancer, I was homeschooling our children. So we did a unit study on the basics of cancer. Weird, right? But it was a great decision. It helped the kids (and me) learn the new vocabulary that we would soon be hearing and using. It helped us all take a step back and treat cancer as a subject, one which could be discussed in a scientific way. In general, it just helped to diffuse some of the emotion and to encourage more analysis — even on an elementary level. It also enabled us to compartmentalize, or set boundaries around, the illness.

Boundaries are important because any major illness tends to engulf your entire life, quickly becoming the soundtrack that plays behind everything you think, say, and do. Gathering information will show you the numbers of people affected by serious diagnoses and the countless variations of these illnesses. That, in turn, can help us to resist the normal tendency to focus on one's self. Studying whatever disease has interrupted your life also empowers you to process the entire situation. Catholicism is known for bringing faith and reason together. Now is a good time to use both of those to the fullest in your own life.

The life you are living at this moment in time, with extra everything — more phone calls, more doctors, different foods, more exhaustion plus the normal requirements of life — is likely to leave you gasping for air. This is true for friends, family members, and caretakers as well. It can feel like a crazy theme park filled with terrifying thrill rides, rollercoaster highs and lows, and lots of screaming — at least internally. In the midst of all this, you need something else, or better yet *someone* else, to focus on.

Finding more time for prayer when you're struggling to squeeze more into your calendar than ever seems almost laughable. However, many will find that they are already praying more than ever before. The trick is to gradually move from constant prayers of desperation to other types of prayer. You can do this slowly and with gentleness. Your prayer does not need to be memorized, scheduled, or regulated. Just as after the initial shock of a serious diagnosis, one moves into acceptance and a new routine, so your prayer life can also move from panic to peace. Reading a sentence like that last one can drive me crazy. The fact is, it's not that easy, and I do not intend to present it as if it is.

When learning to do repetitive 360-degree spins, ballet dancers are taught to focus on one stationery point, just one, while they are spinning. This technique is called spotting, and it is the only way to keep balance and stability. In the same way, you can find more balance in the midst of medical nightmares when you keep a focus, not on yourself but on God. There are many ways to do this — and the more options you can develop, the better.

Be Grateful

A simple place to start is to be grateful. Grateful? This seems counterintuitive at best. What is there to be grateful for when you or a loved one has just received horrible news; maybe even news of a terminal diagnosis? No one is asking you to be happy about what is happening. But you don't have to be *grateful for* your situation to be *grateful in* the challenges you are facing. If you can look around you and find something, anything, that is good, it can change your whole outlook.

In the midst of trying and failing to gain some control of my life after my stage III cancer diagnosis, a dear friend sent me a gift of a blank journal. The short note that came with it simply said to write five things every day for which I was grateful. This was nice. But I cannot say that I appreciated it at first. I had no idea how life changing that small journal would be.

The first few pages of my gratitude journal are blank. Then I wrote Luke 12:4-8:

> I tell you, my friends, do not be afraid of those who kill the body but after that can do no more. I shall show you whom to fear. Be afraid of the one who after killing has the power to cast into Gehenna; yes, I tell you, be afraid of that one. Are not five sparrows sold for two small coins? Yet not one of them has escaped the notice of God. Even the hairs of your head have all been counted. Do not be afraid. You are worth more than many sparrows. I tell you, everyone who acknowledges me before others the Son of Man will acknowledge before the angels of God.

Then more blank pages. Finally, I began and actually made a list of six things for which I was grateful. Then I kind of ruined it with a written rant of self-pity (only one sentence, really) to Jesus. On that first attempt, I started each line with "I am thankful...." My words, when I read them now, sound as if I had to force myself to be thankful for things I know I really did appreciate. Many days it was simple things — a warm house, hearing my kids laugh, sunshine. Other times, I did not have the energy to write even five words. But eventually, almost every night, I managed to add a short list in my gratitude journal.

The result was that during the day, I began to look for good things to be happy about. And you know what? I found them! It is twenty years later, and I am still grateful for those things. Without the gift and encouragement from my friend, I would never have been able to see all the good that was in my life at the time. The lesson of the journal was to look — actively look — for good during a miserable time and to thank God for that good on a daily basis. Writing in it motivated my search and led me in a kind of gentle accountability to God.

We cannot always control what happens in our life, but we can control our attitude toward life. When we start finding the positives, we become more positive ourselves. Give it a try! Caregivers and loved ones can benefit from this just as much as someone who is sick. Make it simple: pen (or pencil) and paper. Start with a list of five things. As you start this simple habit, see where the pen leads — prayers, petitions, outpourings of anger, questions that may only be answered in heaven. You may find that writing can assist you in many ways. Writing allows you to tell your concerns to God at midnight. It can help you process things you may not want to discuss with those closest to you. Writing can release the tears you may choose to bottle up in public. The investment is worth a hundred or thousand times the five dollars and five minutes it will cost you. But don't stress over days you don't write, your penmanship, grammar, spelling, or frustration. Your journal is a no-guilt, no-perfectionism zone. It is just you, pen, and paper. That's it. See where it leads you.

Connect with Jesus

After my chemotherapy failed, I had surgery. As I left the hospital twenty-four hours later, I was handed a sheet of instructions of things that were supposed to have been done within the first twenty-four hours to avoid complications. Just great. I left the hospital with two drains around the incision that removed my breast. Not fun, and yucky to boot. But my sour attitude was soon tempered by an insight I never expected.

Suddenly, I thought of Jesus' crucifixion and remembered a sentence from Saint John's Gospel that "one soldier thrust his lance into his side, and immediately blood and water flowed out" (Jn 19:34). This Bible verse helped to balance me immediately, and in the months thereafter.

It was a grace-filled moment. The realization that Jesus had been through something like what I was experiencing gave it all meaning. It helped me to identify with Jesus on a level I never had been able to do before. My sufferings were nothing compared to his, but now I had something in common with my Savior. Connecting my wounds with his reminded me that it was possible to offer up my sufferings for others, just as Jesus did for me. Remembering what the Son of God endured helped me to look at my own troubles in a different way, a holier way. For me, it was more of a this-is-still-terrible-but-now-it-has-meaning kind of way.

Jesus *wants* to connect with us. I guess I needed something this major to strengthen my connection with him, but that doesn't have to be the case. Hopefully, you are already closer to him than I was. But whether you are or not, know that Jesus is already reaching out to you. If you are suffering mental anguish, think of his agony in the garden the night he was betrayed. If headaches are a problem, reflect on how he was crowned with thorns. If diabetes or neuropathy limits your mobility or increases your risk of falling, contemplate him carrying the cross, uphill, through the rocky streets of Jerusalem. No matter what your ailment or distress, Jesus has gone before you in some way. He is already there waiting for you to join him. When you look for a connection that can bring you closer to him, you will find one.

Trust God

My situation also brought to mind an image of Jesus: The Divine Mercy. This picture is present in many Catholic churches and can easily be found on the internet as well. Devotion to Divine Mercy has spread throughout the world in the past few decades. It began in the 1930s when Jesus appeared to a Polish nun, now Saint Faustina. Jesus instructed her to have someone paint what he revealed. In the image, Jesus is dressed in white with red and white rays of light coming from his heart.

The simplicity of the image allows us to see whatever we need to see in it. For me, at first, it was the red and white rays of grace. For others, it may be his eyes. Later, I noticed how he was taking a step toward the viewer, showing his desire to come to us. There is a set of prayers that can be prayed as a chaplet on rosary beads; a nine-day novena; and the actual diary of Saint Faustina to read. The entire devotion can be boiled down to the image itself and the five words inscribed at the bottom of it: "Jesus, I trust in you."

Those five words are so simple, so beautiful, and so consoling. They are five words to cling to when confronted with heartrending news, or when we feel confused, lonely, or even in despair. Five words that are easy to memorize or say, yet hard to live. There are times when we believe and trust because there is nothing else. That is why the picture shows Jesus taking that step toward us. Because he is the Good Shepherd, Jesus is always looking for us — and inviting us to trust in him.

Let Go of Big Plans

But sometimes with illness that "always" disappears. Sometimes the burden is overwhelming, or all the medication tears your memory away. There was a time when the only words I could remember of the Hail Mary were those first two words: "Hail Mary." That was it; the rest was gone. It made me frustrated and angry, even though I did not have enough energy for those emotions. But as I accepted that those two words were all I had, a peace settled in my soul and reassured me that it was all okay. My plan to pray three Rosaries a day (and try to catch up for years of not saying any) was a no-go. I had seldom taken an over-the-counter pain reliever, and it was obvious that I had grossly underestimated the impact of modern drug therapies.

The thing I finally realized is that neither God nor Mary cares about those details. God is our loving Father. He wants to provide for and protect us. And Mary is our mother — better yet, our mom. She wants to console us and hold our hand and reassure us. She always wants to bring us to her Son and teach us how to have trust in him. So, if the words disappear, don't worry or despair. Hold the image of The Divine Mercy in your mind and just rest in his peace.

So use your fingers on one hand as a reminder to look for and write down five things for which you are grateful. Use the fingers on your other hand to remember the five words, "Jesus, I trust in you." Ten fingers to bring you closer to God. Ten fingers to trust that God can make you the best person you have ever been, even while you are feeling your absolute worst.

Chapter Three

MORE CHANGES

*"Do not let your hearts be troubled.
You have faith in God; have faith also in me."*
— JOHN 14:1

After a period of time, you may be surprised to find that you have some breathing room. A difficult diagnosis will still be able to throw new things in your direction. But the difference is that you won't be caught completely off guard and may have more time between the barrages of new information. Whatever your medical challenges are, you have integrated them into your new reality. Your old routine has been replaced by something that is totally different, but it is slowly becoming a new routine. It's ironic, but this is good, even if you don't like the reason for it one bit!

Routines can become ruts, but it is highly doubtful that your new medical regimen will become one. Enjoy the stability while you can, for things will probably change more quickly than normal life routines before your diagnosis ever would have. And those changes don't just come with declining health. For example, when a prognosis improves, the schedule will change, the treatment type and location may change, and the staff may also change — all from good news!

Who's in Control?

With frequent changes, deeper issues may surface. For many, an underlying desire to control is revealed. Once you enter the medical world with a serious disease or ailment, you are expected to rely on the experts. This is why they — and we — are there after all. It is difficult to recognize that despite lengthy appointments which lay out the options, quite often it doesn't feel like there are any options at all. It's like being given two choices of food, both of which you hate. You aren't going to feel like you a have a choice, even though you do. Often, we do not like the choices we are given simply because we do not like the situation we are in.

Moreover, it can seem that every professional — from financial aid personnel to surgeons — expects you to follow all their recommendations and do what they say, when they say it. The clearly preferred option we are given is often accompanied by some version of all the very bad things that will happen if we choose not to follow it. While the warnings may be true, this kind of interaction with medical professionals negates the sense of having made a choice. It can also make us feel like we are no longer able to exercise even a small amount of control over our own lives. Handling it all can be tricky, especially because, as experts, our health professionals should know what is best for us. While this is normally the case, it is not always true, and the overwhelming tides of emotions, information, and bewildering choices can quickly become a toxic brew.

Dealing with Feelings

The emotions that came with the diagnosis you received (denial, anger, sorrow, etc.) and the emotions that rise from the loss of control (confusion, anger, resentment) need to be addressed in some fashion. When you add the helter-skelter of medical appointments, procedures, plus people that need to be consulted and/or consoled, well, the inside of your head can become a bit of a zoo.

At one point after I was past the initial craziness and in treatment, I asked for a week off from active treatment. One week to clear my mind, sort through the information about possible next steps to take, and just let the mountain of stuff filter, without any new options or treatments or personnel. Depending on what you are dealing with, that may or may not be possible. Perhaps interrupting treatment isn't something that you would even want to consider. In any case, it will be necessary to consult with the physicians involved.

I was told that my request was both unusual and not at all welcome. My doctor did not forbid my "week off," but he made it clear that he wasn't thrilled. So I thought some more, prayed about it, talked to my husband, and ended up deciding to take a week off anyway. I realize there are times you simply *must* proceed with treatment at lightning speed — I already had — and you should obey your doctor's recommendations. When I made this request, however, I was just upsetting the clinic's routine, not courting imminent death.

That week turned out to be a true gift for my mental health. It gave me time to rest from the earlier treatments, and it made my body stronger. It gave me time to set up a plan for my children's schedules while moving forward with my cancer treatment. It gave my husband and me time to reconnect and strengthen our marriage for the unknown challenges ahead. And it gave me time to go and sit in church by myself and begin a change: a change from talking *to* God to talking *with* God.

When I returned to the clinic the following week, my doctor asked if I had enjoyed my "vacation." Smiling, I told him it was great. He remained silent but took a good long look at me. Then he "harrumphed," gave a tiny smile, and we got back to work and back to the plan.

I am not recommending that you delay urgent treatment or pick a fight with your doctor. What I am saying is that if you feel like the rollercoaster is about to throw you off into the ocean, please talk to your team of medical professionals and ask them to help you find some time to rest and think. A brief time off may be possible at some point, and it cannot hurt to ask.

Talking with God

Whether or not you are able to take a short break from the whirlwind, try to switch from talking at God, or to God, to talking *with* him. For me, this change was very gradual and very fruitful. The more I took time to talk with God, the more I felt his presence at other times. The more I felt his presence, the more I wanted to talk with him. Just remember that in a conversation one has to leave pauses to let the other person speak. For me, it took some time before I could even think to leave space for him. I would go before the Eucharist at my parish and spend the whole time uploading all my troubles to God — repeatedly — and not even remembering to leave silence for him to speak.

If treatment gets rougher and when the reality of changed circumstances sets in, these silent conversations become more and more important. But you do not need to be in a church. Time in the hospital is a great opportunity to visit with the Lord too. After all, Jesus went about healing the sick, and that included talking with them.

A waiting room or doctor's office may have too many distractions and too many different people. But waiting rooms are places that make it easy to remember to pray for others. All you have to do is look around the room and pray for those you see around you. Silently ask God to give hope to others. I learned this from a fellow chemo patient. She somehow recognized me as another Catholic and asked if I had prayed the Sacred Heart Novena. When I replied that I had not, she said that I just had to have it. The next day, she brought me a black-and-white copy of her favorite prayer, carefully glued together and trimmed. I still have that holy card many years later, and I still pray it. It's a visible reminder of a fellow patient's act of kindness.

The change from talking "to" God to "with" God was also the beginning of my giving up ultimate control, at least to God. Now, of course, God is *always* in control, and always has been. That does not mean that we suddenly stop telling him what his plan *should* be. The medical crisis you are facing was probably not in your plan. The simple answer to moving forward is to give it all over to God. Immediately. I wish I could write that I did all these things myself. I can't. But, as Saint Paul wrote in Romans 7:19: "For I do not do the good I want, but I do the evil I do not want." Try not to fret or become discouraged, but just keep giving all your concerns and all your regrets over your "lost plan" back to God. And realize that it may take some time.

What Gives You Peace?

Look for things that give you peace. On the physical, human level it may be a cup of tea, a flower, a favorite picture, or a small tabletop fountain. The point is to surround yourself with things that help you relax. For some, activity brings peace. If you aren't feeling up to things you've enjoyed in the past, try reading, listening to music, or simple handcrafts. Now there are even coloring books for adults! When we are able to relax, we become more able to communicate with God. We also become more able to heal.

Just as looking for things to write in my gratitude journal encouraged me to look for those things, speaking with God encouraged me to look for peace-giving things in my surroundings. For example, as spring arrived, I was desperate for flowers: seeds to plant in the garden; flowers to plant by the house; fresh flowers for my bedroom, where I needed to rest for hours. Maybe your taste is more for a beautiful picture, photographs of the people you love, or Scripture verses written in gorgeous calligraphy. If it reminds you of God, and gives you peace, use it.

Accept God's Gifts

Everything from a great parking spot to a sunny day is a gift from God. Allow these things to bring you joy. Yes, even when you are in the most difficult times of your life, you are still capable of feeling joy. When things go wrong, as they will some days, thank God and ask him to take whatever went wrong or the bad news or the lousy day and turn it into something beautiful. It still may not be beautiful for you, but maybe it will be for someone else. And ask him to keep any losses or negative feelings from spilling over into another day.

To look for gifts in daily life is to find gifts in daily life. If you let it, serious illness will help you re-focus on things we all miss in everyday life because we are caught up in busyness and routines. The changed circumstances forced by a serious illness gives you the opportunity to intently focus on finding beauty and good wherever you are. Living with a serious diagnosis is usually both high speed and slow as molasses. Train yourself to look for the good at both paces.

Nature, God's creation, can also be a big help. After trips to the doctor, I made a point of sitting in the car to watch the Missouri River flow by. Some days, the river seemed lazy. Other days, whirlpools would spin and disappear quickly. After heavy rains, whole trees would be frantically floating downstream. I longed for the lazy, sunny river but knew that for this season of my life, I was dealing with whirlpools and destroyed trees. Knowing that allowed me to realize that the calm would come; I just had to wait for it and endure the tree branches in the meantime.

Find somewhere accessible to nature where you can sit and enjoy the view. Cities and towns are very accommodating, with wheelchair-accessible paths and even fishing docks. If you have trouble thinking of a place to go, ask God to show you one where you can find some peace. While you're at it, ask him to provide a nice day and a ride as well. Then watch what happens!

If possible, plan ahead for any hospital stays and ask for a room with a view. It may not be available, but you can ask. If friends wonder what they can do, consider asking them to bring fresh flowers or a plant once in a while, especially while you're hospitalized. God wants us to enjoy his creation. We need it, just like we need him.

Inner Peace

Even more important is peace on the spiritual level. I'm convinced that the best, easiest, and most portable way to peace wherever you are is to pray the Rosary. It takes about fifteen minutes, and it will give you peace. You do not need to be Catholic to pray the Rosary. It is simply repeated prayers, or "roses," offered to Mary, the Mother of Jesus. The Rosary is an ancient form of meditation that helps people to focus on events in the life of Jesus through a series of "mysteries." People have prayed it for centuries, not only to bring themselves peace but also as a way to bring peace to others, and even to the world.

Perhaps you don't remember how to pray the Rosary, and maybe you aren't sure where to find the set of rosary beads that someone once gave you. This is not a problem. Mention wanting a rosary to almost anyone, Catholic or not, and I bet you will have a free one within a day. If you are unable to speak, just silently ask the Virgin Mary or Jesus and, trust me, one will show up. Praying the Rosary is not hard, and there are countless media resources to help, including online instructions and audio recordings. The Rosary is even prayed on television, radio, and live on Facebook! For many people, the rhythm of familiar words like those in the Our Father and the Hail Mary provides a comfortable place for prayer to begin.

Make Friends with the Saints

For additional spiritual peace, consider looking to the saints for consolation and guidance. There are so many wonderful men and women of faith who can bring us closer to God and who can become our friends in heaven. Read about the saint of the day with an app, website, or book. If one particular saint strikes a chord with you, read more about that person. Think about how that saint might have reacted had he or she been in your situation. What was that saint's fears or weaknesses? How did he or she overcome those obstacles?

Allow yourself to be inspired by the lives of these holy people. And do so knowing that most of them didn't start out holy! Sometimes, during serious, especially long-term diagnosis living, we cannot help but be alone physically and emotionally, so cultivating a friendship with the saints is a true lifeline, in more ways than one.

Chapter Four

SURRENDER

"It is the LORD who goes before you; he will be with you and will never fail you or forsake you. So do not fear or be dismayed."
— DEUTERONOMY 31:8

Somewhere along the way, in the back of your mind, come questions about how you are going to treat what you are facing from a mental or almost philosophical perspective. This is seldom, if ever, discussed. When you're confronted with a major medical diagnosis, physical needs take immediate priority, and turning inward is natural. If, however, you begin to close yourself off to others or obsess exclusively on the illness, it's time to re-evaluate or consider talking with someone.

A Broader View

With some diseases, "focusing on yourself" is actively encouraged. This is not as bad as it sounds, as each of us is encouraged to take care of our bodies as gifts from God. But we should always be aware that, while necessary, the focus on self should not be long term. I was actually pitied by many people for having young children, not because it was possible *they* would lose their mother, but because *I* would be unable to focus completely on myself. The fact that my children kept me from thinking only about what was wrong with me is something I'm still thankful for. I also attended a cancer support group. I stopped going after a few months when I realized that for many of the group's members, cancer had become the sole focus of their daily lives. *Everything* was about cancer.

So how can your life include more than just the illness you or your loved one is facing?

The first step is the decision to surrender your situation to God. In other words, to accept God's will for you, at this point in time. I love holy writers who illustrate and encourage the right movements toward God. But I am a person who screws it all up, takes one step forward and three back, and wants visible results — immediately. The lesson for me was that I needed to stop telling God what he *should* do and surrender to what God *was doing*. Even deeper, I needed to personally surrender myself, and not just my illness, to him.

Choose Your Battles

But surrender? That seems like such a terrible word! John Wayne never surrendered! Or maybe he did. This is an instance in which the word itself is the problem, especially when our culture and healthcare professionals encourage us to "fight." You may choose to fight your disease or illness. But you must not fight God's will. So somehow, you have to find a mental place where you can separate the two. It is not impossible to do this, but people tend to lose sight of it. Once again, the shock and rapidity of treatments can tend to draw you away from God when you need him most. Do not let this happen.

The reality is that without surrendering to God, life can be lonely. Whether sick or healthy, young or old, only God can constantly be with us. Only God knows everything we need. Only God completely understands who we are. Surrender is almost always considered "bad," but if that surrender is to God and his will, it can only be good!

Giving It Up Isn't Giving Up

When you surrender to God, you don't suddenly become the star in a sad movie that ends in despair and humiliation. Surrendering your circumstances and your life to God is a beautiful lifting up of all you are to the one who loves you most of all, best of all, and forever. It is not a hunkering down, depressive zone at all.

You probably have anticipated God's plan and have it all laid out in front of you. But you don't actually know what his will is for you tomorrow — only for today. The future is always unknown, and the unknown is always frightening. That just feeds into our fear of what might happen if we turn our lives over to God. If you can focus on accepting what you face today as God's will, you will see the fear begin to disappear.

When you choose to surrender to God, the result is joy, lightness, and relief. Joy that God, who we know loves us, is in control. Lightness in that much of the responsibility has been lifted from our shoulders (and our blood pressure) and given to God. Relief that someone is going to stay with us and work with us in our pains and sufferings now, and in the future. Even better, we also know that this someone has lived similar pains and sufferings: he understands us totally. Now that we have handed over our troubles to the one who can actually do something with those troubles, we can breathe more calmly.

Loved ones and caregivers also struggle with surrender. No one plans for a friend or family member to become ill. Surrendering to God's plan can sometimes even be a greater mountain to climb for those who love the patient, than for the patient themselves. Gentleness — and trust — are needed by all involved, with one another, and with God.

The Struggle to Trust

This refusal to surrender our lives to God is usually based on fear: fear that God will not do what we ask. In all honesty, he may not. But there is also the underlying idea that only I know what *should* happen. That isn't fear but rather an I-know-best (better-than-God) attitude. The sad thing is that when we struggle against God in a difficult time, it is often just at the point when he is ready to pour out graces in abundance.

Like forgiveness, surrendering your life to God may take more than one attempt. In fact, it may take years or even a lifetime. Keep asking God for the grace to lean on him and to trust in him. I still ask God to remind me to surrender to him. That's because my personal character traits (doesn't that sound much better than "my faults"?) almost guarantee that I will, within a short time, be running off in the wrong direction.

Mental Approach

Thinking about how to approach your illness mentally is another part of the challenge. Many cancer patients choose an almost military strategy against cancer, and it is successful for a lot of them. I thought it was a good plan myself. Yet it bothered me that the cancer cells were mine and that most people have cancer cells that are kept under control by their bodies. For whatever reason, my body could not (or did not) keep them under control. I did not want to focus on killing cancer cells but rather on encouraging my "helper" cells to surround and calm my cancer cells so they would stop reproducing.

Eventually, my approach evolved into accepting whatever God allowed. Not only the treatment but also the cancer itself. In any case, it is helpful to think about how *you* want to approach whatever you may be coping with. Decide how you are going to handle dialysis or physical therapy or weekly chemo. That choice is an individual one. You may want to discuss this with your loved ones as well so that they can model or reflect back your chosen approach when you need support on down days. Remember, too, that an approach can be changed. Nothing you decide about how to handle your challenge is written in stone. If you find it less than helpful, try something else.

Shared Burdens

It's important to remember, too, that our own suffering can and usually does trigger suffering for others. At home for four days between treatments, my youngest daughter woke up crying in the night. I went to her and asked her what was wrong, thinking it was a nightmare. She said, "I'm tired of you being sick!"

It was a nightmare — for all of us! A day later, I was playing with my three-year-old son and the game was "Let's take Mama to the doctor!" I tried to convince myself that it was a sign that he was coping well with everything we were going through as a family, but it was not the game I wanted to be playing with my son.

Your illness, whatever it is, affects not only you and your direct caregiver. Your attitude and choice of how to mentally approach being sick also affects those you know and love. This includes not only your closest relatives but also coworkers, neighbors, and fellow parishioners. Your choices, your actions, and your words have significant — and potentially positive! — impact on them.

Chapter Five

SUBMISSION

*David answered Gad: "I am greatly
distressed. But let us fall into the hand
of God, whose mercy is great...."*
— 2 SAMUEL 24:14

It took me a while to figure out that surrender wasn't the same as submission. I didn't have to just stop fighting God's will; I had to choose to actively live it out. That put a real wrench into my plans.

Do What Is Possible

When I entered the hospital for the second time, I went in with a plan for Bible reading, Rosaries, and favorite prayers, despite my favorite priest's reminders to "rest in the Lord" and to simply surrender myself to God. He was so much wiser than I was. I soon found that with the medicines I was given, none of my intense spiritual "agenda" was possible. At times, I offered it all up to God. I tried to make my own version of the Morning Offering. There was no way I could remember the prayer, which I had had memorized since childhood, and my eyes were temporarily affected by the chemo, so reading was difficult. In addition, I could not concentrate well at all. Father's admonition to "rest in the Lord" was excellent advice, and most of the time it was the only choice as well.

Tie Your Suffering to Someone Else's

After a while, I learned to make what I call "relational" prayers. I do not mean prayers for your relations, although that is a great thing too. Rather, I tried to relate, or tie, my suffering to the suffering of others. If sick to my stomach, I would pray for those who were nauseous or for pregnant moms with morning sickness. If I was horribly hungry but could not eat, I would pray for hungry people around the world. If sleep eluded me, I would pray for those going to work in China. (I had actually started doing this when I was up with kids and, resentfully, did not want to pray for any lucky person on my side of the world who was still asleep. A very bad attitude on my part!)

Receiving shots became a time to pray for drug addicts, and receiving blood transfusions (which totally freaked me out) meant prayers for whoever donated the blood. On really bad days, when I was the center of a pity party in full swing, the grace of God would remind me to pray for those being tortured in dark prisons around the world. Eventually, I realized that it was a perfect time for a hospital version of Eucharistic Adoration. Right in the isolation room.

These prayers never took long, nor were they formal. The *Catechism of the Catholic Church* states that prayer is simply "the raising of one's mind and heart to God or the requesting of good things from God" (CCC 2559). In my feeble way, that's what I was trying to do. All these "relational" prayers were simple attempts to use my suffering for someone else's benefit. If what I was experiencing could be offered as a sacrifice to God along with my prayers, my part of the conversation with God would be more powerful than just words alone. These prayers will be different from day to day and also from person to person. Just begin, and remember that to God everything counts.

Answers to Prayer

Can I prove that any of these prayers "worked"? No, but I believe they did, some in ways that I will not know about until I (hopefully!) reach heaven. But I do know that praying helped me in many ways. Prayer took me out of myself and directed me toward others, especially when the temptation to make my life all about me and me alone was at its strongest. Also, the prayers I offered for the world reminded me that there was, in fact, a world outside the hospital. Being mindful of others' needs kept me in touch with the truth that things can almost always be worse than they are, even worse than a bad medical diagnosis.

Choices

My second round of chemo began immediately after rush surgery, but it still didn't work. That was obviously not good news. My oncologist then referred me to an uber-oncologist who recommended a stem cell transplant. His plan for me was regular chemo while I recovered from surgery, followed by a higher dose of chemo. Then, he would harvest my own stem cells and freeze them. After giving me a super-high dose of chemo that would take me near death, he would thaw my stem cells and put them back into my body. The process required months in an isolation unit located in a large city an hour away. If I survived all that, I could recuperate and then begin daily radiation treatments.

It didn't take me long to say, "No thanks." And when everyone else told me I had to do it — my husband, doctors, relatives, and friends — I still said no. It was not so much fear of the treatments (though I was afraid), or even fear of death (because that was in the mix either way). It was that I did not want to be separated from my children. They would not have been able to visit, and I would not see them for months. At this point, I knew how fragile I was emotionally. To me, a forced separation like this would kill me in a way I could not imagine coming back from. Ever. My husband asked if I would at least pray about it. Reluctantly, I said I would.

Signs

So, I said some very "bad" prayers. I told God I did not want to do this, had no intention of doing it, and was going to make it hard on him (hah!) by asking for a sign. I gave him from Friday until Monday to send me roses, but not just any roses. Saint Thérèse of Lisieux is famous for sending roses from heaven, and Saint Maximilian Kolbe chose both the white crown of purity and the red crown of martyrdom offered to him by the Virgin Mary. I combined both of these favorite saints' histories with a demand (it should have been a request, but in all honesty, it was a demand) for both red and white roses. I told absolutely no one about the "one time offer" I was making to God.

"On paper." These two words popped into my head immediately. I paused and thought, well, I guess paper roses would count and gave a silent mental consent to paper roses or roses on paper, thinking that might even be more difficult than real flowers. The fact was that I had other things to think about. My husband was shaving my hair off that night. It had been coming out in huge clumps, sometimes unexpectedly, so it was time. He was also cutting the boys' hair to the same length — i.e., a boot camp buzz. We exempted the girls, of course, but their Aunt Pat had made them matching pink polka dot scarves, which they would wear to the shaving party. Afterward, we watched television and had snacks. Just another fun Friday night with cancer.

The next day, my friend Lois dropped by. She just wanted to say hello and drop off some magazines for me. She had brought some a week or two before and had found another one lodged in a drawer where she was sure she had looked earlier. No big deal — it gave her a reason to stop by and check out my new un-hair style. We were visiting at the kitchen table when I stopped listening. There, in the magazine she had just said shouldn't have been where it was, was a full color, half-page spread of roses. Red roses, white roses, yellow roses, peach roses. On paper. The day after I issued my demand to God.

I wish I could say that I told her immediately, hugged her, and thanked her for being a true messenger from heaven. Being a total stinker, I said nothing, finished the visit, and tried to ignore the photo. Which was impossible, of course. Hours went by. My husband asked if I had prayed. Yes. Did I have any signs? I refused to answer. That's how he knew.

Submission

A day or two later, I wrote a thank-you note to Saint Max and Saint Thérèse in my journal. God had given me the sign I had asked for, and within twenty-four hours at that. It obviously meant that I should accept the treatment recommendation. I truly was thankful for the roses because it made my path clear. But I cannot say that it made me joyful. My journal contained a note of gratitude for those praying for me, but it was also a big bite of humility regarding my own rebelliousness and ingratitude.

Surrendering to God was one thing, but submitting to the Lord's will when it so directly opposed mine was another. Some people seem graced with the ability to submit to God's will with joy immediately. But for me it was a battle. I asked my pastor to send me a list of prayers or a list of Scripture readings. He refused and told me that my focus should be my acceptance of God's will for me and obedience to that will. I was to constantly surrender myself and my situation to God: to put it all in God's hands. This was more difficult than any reading or prayer assignment he could have given me. I was not a fan. That same week, a friend suggested a radio program she liked. When I turned it on, it was all about surrendering your situation to God. God has a sense of humor.

For me, submission was not a one-time act because I kept taking it back. I had to submit to the Lord daily, at times even hourly. Saints tell us that's how we should live, but I needed to learn to live that way — and with a much better attitude. Saint Paul once healed a man who had never walked, because he saw that the man "had the faith to be healed" (see Acts 14:8–10). One of my prayers at the time was to have that kind of faith: the faith to trust, to believe, and to be made well. Gradually, it also became a prayer for the kind of faith I needed to accept God's will — whatever that would be — with joy and love.

Chapter Six

NORMAL

"Be still and know that I am God!"
— PSALM 46:11

"I just want to go home and be normal again."

I remember writing that in my journal. The initial panic had subsided, choices had been made, treatments were on-going, and now there was a space of time to think. The re-sult was sadness and depression. The gratitude list was gone, saints seemed to be hiding, God was silent, and I was not allowed visitors.

The desire to be "normal" again comes and goes throughout any illness. On some level, we all want the sim-plicity of a normal life at home. The routines we used to fret about, or even resent, we may dream of now. But life chang-es for many reasons and so can we. Few want to think of serious illness as a part of normal life, but in many ways it is. For some, struggling with this will be a big issue; for others, it may not be an issue at all. Neither is right or wrong — it is just that people are different, sick or not. Regardless of those many differences, however, everyone wants to feel at home.

Distant from God

Even if we've considered ourselves close to God, it can seem as if he disappears into thin air when life is shaken by a major illness or condition. The truth is that we may not really know how close we are to God in any circumstance. We do know, though, that God wants to be close to us. It is important, therefore, to admit that distance from God may be the consequence of our choice to keep him at a distance. If so, now is the time to reconnect.

But what if you don't *want* to reconnect? What if you are still angry? These feelings are real and can belong to pa-tients, caregivers, loved ones, or even coworkers or friends as well. So, first, tell God you are angry. You may even want to tell him that you don't want to talk to him. By doing so, you are relieving some of your own anger, tension, and resentment — but also recognizing his existence. That is a starting point.

Second, think about people who have nothing. It seems cliché but not if you really consider how little some people have and yet are still able to live with exuberant joy and love for God.

Third, read the Bible story of the Prodigal Son in Luke 15:11–32. Most people know the basic plot line, but try looking at it from the point of view of each of the different characters. The father was not treated fairly by the son who couldn't even wait for him to die to get his money; the older brother kept working while his younger brother was partying, which was not fair to him; and the prodigal son, who "should" have been disowned, was greeted with open arms instead. Not fair all around. But it all turned right with the father's love. What do you think could happen if you dared God to show you that he cared? Why not find out?

God Is Near

As Christians, we believe that God is near. You may not realize it, but during this time of illness God is closer than ever. Then why doesn't it feel that way?

Imagine that you are having a great time swimming ten yards out from shore in the ocean. The shore does not seem that far away; it's an easy swim. But add a shark to the scene and the ten yards to shore seems impossibly far away. If you focus on getting to shore and *stay* focused on getting to shore, the odds are in your favor because the shore is close. But if you focus on the shark instead, and spend your time thrashing around and screaming, you may not even know where the shore is, let alone make it in time. When we or someone we care about is suddenly confronting danger, we lose our bearings. It's easy to forget that God is *not* the shark. God is the safe, warm, welcoming shore.

God is always here for us. He can provide us a feeling of "home" wherever we are. That's because God is our ultimate home. Saint Augustine said, "Our hearts are restless, O Lord, until they rest in you." If we focus only on fear, pain, and possible negative outcomes, everything becomes more difficult. But if, during the challenging times of a serious diagnosis, we can learn to focus on God, everything becomes healthier and more positive. Living your new normal improves when you get closer to God.

Move Closer to God

Because God is near, getting closer to him is easy. Honestly, we don't even have to do much. How about saying "Good morning" to God? That takes about two seconds. As you get comfortable with that, tell him what you are concerned about for the day. After a few days, add in a prayer or two for someone else who has a problem; if you don't know of anyone in particular, count your blessings and thank him for them. The possibilities are truly endless!

Am I saying the hospital or the dialysis clinic will feel just like home? Of course not. Hopefully, though, you will become at least a little bit friendly with staff and fellow patients. In any case, pray for them. If that still seems too lofty or difficult, just think of all the people who need prayers but have no one to pray for them. Now may be your chance to offer your own fear, discomfort, and pain for others like you have never done before. This will help you transition to a new normal.

When You're Down

Whatever settings you are led to through your illness, remember that there will be people there who need your help and consolation. But sometimes it is necessary to deal with your own emotions before you can do anything else. Do not add feeling bad about feeling bad to your list of troubles.

If you have to — or need to — have a pity-party or a good long cry, do it! But end it when the sun goes down so that you have time to settle your heart. The psalms in the Bible are full of emotional pleas. Search through the Book of Psalms to find one that matches how you are feeling. Or you can just open your Bible to Psalms (almost always right in the center) and ask the Holy Spirit to point out the right psalm for you. You may also discover a few of God's promises to read during these troubling times. Some especially good ones include Psalms 4, 6, 103, 116, 130, 138, and 142.

When the next day dawns, you will be refreshed and able to be on the lookout for others who are not even as strong as you are and who need your help. Let the Lord lead you and strengthen you.

Go Beyond Just You

Don't be surprised if the Lord puts other people on your path, such as other patients or their caregivers. Just try to be positive and encouraging when you encounter them. Be aware that it is not always fellow patients who need encouragement. Doctors, nurses, receptionists, and cleaning personnel all bear their own crosses; questions or comments can and do come from anyone.

A friend of a friend, used to say, "If I have to go to the hospital, then that means someone needs to hear about Our Lord." I am not one to talk about God or religion much to anyone except my own family. To be honest, I am not that comfortable even writing about this stuff. But strange as it sounds, God sent people to my isolation room who wanted, or needed, to talk. I often had my Bible out and my rosary on my food tray, not because I was waiting to evangelize but because I couldn't move much.

I honestly do not know why this happened. In any case, there are many hurting people in this world who have struggles much deeper than illness or disease. After a long conversation with a nurse, it became clear she was being manipulated by two relatives. Another nurse used to come in and talk about the problems she was having with her children. One of the doctors would go over all the doctor questions and then ask if he could just sit and watch TV with me for a while if it was on. I thought this was strange but noticed he was more relaxed when he left. Saint Paul puts it beautifully:

> Blessed be the God and Father of our Lord
> Jesus Christ, the Father of compassion and
> God of all encouragement, who encour-

ages us in our every affliction, so that we
may be able to encourage those who are
in any affliction with the encouragement
with which we ourselves are encouraged by
God. For as Christ's sufferings overflow to
us, so through Christ does our encouragement also overflow. (2 Cor 1:3–5)

Television

The television is something that remains "normal" in this
time when almost everything else is not. Usually, televisions
are present in all settings: waiting rooms, clinics, hospitals,
and many doctor offices. Television may seem a strange tool
for dealing with medical issues, but it can have a huge effect
on your spiritual and emotional well-being.

I grew up watching television like the rest of my peers.
Lots of hours in front of the screen over the years. Then,
when our children were very small, my husband and I gave
TV up for Lent, and shortly after Easter we went back to
regular consumption. The next Lent, we gave it up again
and stuck with no television for ten years. Yes, ten years. We
did watch the Olympics once or twice, got it out of the closet (literally) for coverage of the terrorist attacks of 9/11, and
also when five of our six kids came down with chicken pox
on Easter Sunday one year. It was back in the closet when I
was diagnosed with cancer.

Television shows can be a familiar "face" in new surroundings, and they can bring a sense of normality to
wherever your illness takes you. Enjoying a favorite show
can bring joy and laughter, which is great. Concentrating

on solving a mystery along with a favorite television sleuth can give your mind a healthy break from worries and treatments. Television shows can also be a topic of conversation that is not medical in nature — also a good thing. But don't forget to leave time for silence.

Find Silence

Everyone needs silence, but most especially those who are grappling with a serious diagnosis. We need time to let the brain rest from the constant noise of our world. Still, anyone who visits hospital patients as an extraordinary minister of Holy Communion will tell you that it is the norm to find the television on, and it is seldom that a television is turned off when they arrive with the Eucharist. Our culture seems to fear silence. But how will we ever hear God if we always surround ourselves with noise?

In some clinics, the television is impossible to escape. The way of least resistance is to just enjoy it, and there is nothing wrong with that. My preference, however, would be to read a book while waiting in public places. Often, though, the television is so obtrusively loud or large that concentrating on a book is impossible.

Though most would expect otherwise, noise often *increases* upon entering intensive care units or during medical procedures. Despite being warned by a kindly nurse, our first experience of the neonatal unit our first child required was overwhelming. There were bright overhead lights, buzzers, alarms, breathing machines and multicolored lights on monitors of all sizes and shapes.

No matter the unit, give yourself time to get used to all the buzzers, alarms, sounds, and motions. Consider letting go of some voluntary screen time. Give yourself and your caregivers quiet to recover from all the stress that noise inflicts on us.

Be Open

When I went into isolation, it seemed like the television was always staring at me. There was not much else I could do, as drugs often impaired my ability to read and visitors were infrequent. But with ten years of abstinence from television, I wasn't sure how to approach it. Often I found the shows annoying.

Two channels and one video became my mainstays. I watched a local channel once in a while, but regular shows were too difficult for me if they had long plot lines. The outdoor channel was a favorite as it brought back memories of trout fishing with my dad. Any time I could find a show with running rivers and streams I counted it as a gift from God. I also had one video of Celtic dance that always brought good energy into the room. Nurses would often take the time to finish watching the song or dance that was playing and went away looking happier. This all happened in an isolation room. If you are up to it, just ask God to help those with whom you will come into contact. Then watch and see what happens.

A month-long stay in an isolation room is a long way from anyone's normal. So, my prayer for home and normality was, technically, not answered. At least, not in the way I desired. Instead, I learned that God could use me for others' good. Not only that, but he could still manage to do this while I was vomiting, bald, and totally isolated except for staff and infrequent, well-scrubbed visitors. How awesome is that! Graces are everywhere if we just ask and then look. It was not home, it was not normal, but it was amazing!

God Is Still with You

Wanting comfort, and waiting for it while suffering, is not easy. It may even be more difficult for those who must watch you suffer. When you're in the midst of it, the chance of going home or getting back to normal may seem even further away than it did the day before. For me, there were days when any movement I made caused me to vomit. And by movement, I mean something as tiny as stretching a foot that was cramping. There were times I could do absolutely nothing. Movement was impossible, talking was impossible, thinking was impossible. You may experience times like that too. I hope not.

But when you are certain that there is nothing left, you will discover that God is still there with you — you might even feel that, somehow, he was there *before* you. Finding God may not change your circumstance, but finding him does change everything else. Mostly, it changes us. God is there for us, if we just look.

A Heavenly Mother

If God seems too distant or too big, you can try asking Jesus' mother, the Blessed Virgin Mary, to sit with you by your bedside. As Catholics, we have a rich tradition of calling on

Mary. From the cross, Jesus said, "Behold, your mother" (Jn 19:27). Jesus was speaking not only to his beloved disciple, John, but to all of us. Mary will be a mother to you as well, if you allow her to be.

Remember back when you were a child and miserable with a fever or the flu. With or without your mother present, you were miserable, but somehow you felt better when she was there. For us, as adults, those days may seem long gone, until illness strikes and then the longing for someone to offer us a wet washcloth or a gentle pat on the hand is overwhelming. Mary listens, she calms, and she prays with us and for us. And even more, Mary always brings us to her son, Jesus. Lean on her and ask for her help whenever you need consolation.

Small Favors Bring Big Blessings

If possible, consider asking one of your friends or relatives to do something small for you. People really do want to help, though it is humbling for us to ask them. Sometimes we are so independent that we forget that those who help us will receive grace. Why not give others the chance to be good?

Spread joy and blessings from your hospital bed by asking for a special treat or favorite drink that you cannot get in the hospital, a holy card that you can look at throughout the day, or a pair of cozy socks. Help others by humbly asking for their assistance in building up your hope. Normal life may seem far off for now, but a little reminder from home can make it feel much closer.

Chapter Seven

TRACKS OF TRUST

Trust in the LORD with all your heart,
on your own intelligence do not rely;
In all your ways be mindful of him,
and he will make straight your paths.
Do not be wise in your own eyes,
fear the LORD and turn away from evil;
This will mean health for your flesh
and vigor for your bones.
— PROVERBS 3:5–8

Medical journeys begin with questions of diagnosis and treatment. But they don't end there. At one point, while trying to write a gratitude list, my handwriting went from normal to erratic. The last legible words that day were "This is ridiculous. It's 9:00 a.m., and I'm going back to bed." It wasn't really going *back* to bed, as I had never left the hospital bed in the first place. But isn't that an allegory for life? You are going along, not perfect but doing okay, making a little progress here and there, and then discover your life has gone completely off the tracks. Any serious diagnosis can throw you — and your loved ones — off the tracks.

My grandfather was a railroad yardmaster for decades. As children, we went to a park where there was a railroad engine he had worked with for years before they were both retired. Grandpa loved trains, and he would ride the trains whenever he got the chance. But he also recognized the dangers of working there and the accidents that could happen in the blink of an eye. That's why the phrase "going off the tracks" was part of our family's vocabulary. It could apply to an actual train accident, a wayward relative, or even a politician who went a few steps too far. It was never a good thing.

A major illness can make us feel as if our lives have gone off the tracks. While not what anyone would call a good thing, these times can be strangely beneficial for us and, sometimes, even turned around. Just like when a wayward relative goes off the tracks, change is possible. Prayers are called for, contacts are made, and creative attempts to solve an impossible human situation can bear fruit. But even if they don't produce the result we hope for, they are, in and of themselves, good. Prayer, community, and problem solving are helpful for illness as well, whether or not the sick person is cured.

Prepare for the Truth

With any major illness, it is important to be honest, at least with yourself. But know that you will hear all kinds of technical terminology and euphemisms for bad news. Medical personnel keep things limited, comprehensible, and calm. That doesn't mean that you cannot ask hard questions and expect answers. Before asking those questions, though, make sure that you are prepared for what you may hear and truly want to know the answers.

Getting medical information in small doses can be a very good thing. After all, at first there is the diagnosis, then the new vocabulary, often followed by scary options. So, it might not be the best idea to request the whole story in one fell swoop. The doctors and nurses realize that, and they are trained to take it slow. Remember that what you are facing may become a more-than-full-time job, and that no one learns a whole new job in one day.

Try to understand where the medical staff is coming from and respect their possible reluctance to answer some of your questions directly. They are usually trying to protect you and your loved ones. If you disagree with that approach, say so, but be polite. The medical staff is trying their best to figure out what kind of information you as an individual want and need. That is not on your chart or lab tests. Some people do not want to know much; others want every detail. You may choose to persist in asking, or ask the same question again on another day or ask another staff person. Or you may choose to wait and not ask for more information than you are given.

Nobody Knows Everything

Recognize, too, that no one will have all the answers. I am always somewhat relieved when I meet an "expert" in any field who admits that they do *not* have an answer to a question. Hopefully, it means that they are honest, at least a little humble, and willing to look things up if they do not know the answers. All of these are good things. Also realize that members of the medical staff are human and have their own stressors, private challenges, and personal baggage like everyone else in this vale of tears. Having said all that, for me, clarity in regard to treatment plans and side effects was a necessity, not an option. Hence, my preference for "off the tracks" instead of "derailment."

Knowledge Isn't Always Power

But remember, even if you get all the clarity you desire, going off the tracks is still possible. That is just life sometimes. We may know everything about our situation and still not be able to do much to change it. If you feel yourself going way off the tracks, whether from anger or sadness or just from being overwhelmed, ask for help. These kinds of feelings may come at any point in the journey, and they need to be addressed. Asking for a chaplain or counselor to help you is often a good idea. That is because the family members and friends you might otherwise rely on may also be struggling to process what is happening to you.

The knowledge and skill your medical team has, as well as the treatment they recommend and provide, may not work for you. In our overly litigious society, we often look for someone to blame when medical intervention or treatment doesn't go as hoped. If the goal of a formal complaint is to make sure a heinous behavior does not happen again, that is one thing. If it is an attempt to get even in some monetary way, well, that is a different kettle of fish. Pray about how you want to use the time and energy you have.

Involve God

Keeping God beside you at every step is not only the best way to survive the journey; it is the only way to *redeem* the journey. This means involving God in both the questions and the answers. Growing closer to God does not mean that you are guaranteed to be healed. His ways are not our ways, after all. All of us, sick or not, are working out our own spiritual redemption, and walking our own path to heaven. If you focus on that, you will bring others along and aid in their journeys. So how can you redeem a time of major illness?

If you have read this far, you know that it starts with a simple decision to invite God to go along with you. That one choice will make all the difference. Then, just take the steps that seem easiest, the baby steps. Anyone can begin by simply talking *to* God. He is big enough to take your anger and fear, and he is strong enough to give you hope in the midst of what you are facing. Then move toward talking *with* God. For Catholics, the available helps are numerous. Depending on where you are in your faith, options can include sacramental confession, a morning offering, Mass, Scripture reading, the Rosary, and many other devotions. The goal is to become closer and closer to God as treatment progresses and as life continues to move forward. That closeness is something you will never lose, regardless of any other loss your illness might bring.

Involving God in the questions, answered or not, though, is essential, for only God can lead us to peace. Peace is a wonderful thing to find in life, but it is especially valuable while you are facing a major medical crisis. There is so much that neither you nor your loved ones can control. Trusting in God helps.

Review Your Life

Once you know that you have put yourself into God's hands, you will be able to face your prognosis and all its possible outcomes. For some, a serious diagnosis may end up being a relatively minor glitch in life. For others, it may be a big question mark or a very long struggle. There will be those, too, for whom it is a terminal diagnosis. Most will find themselves mentally bouncing between those possibilities. But for all of us, medical challenges can offer an important opportunity for introspection. A review of your life is in order.

In a way, this is similar to the familiar New Year's resolutions that we may make. But with a major diagnosis, this life review takes on a new seriousness that those end-of-December reviews never had. No matter what your past has been, the questions pop up in great number — especially those having to do with your illness: *Will I be able to stick with exercising? Can I really stop smoking? Can I control my weight? Give up my soda addiction? Who will raise my children*

*if things get worse? Will Aunt Hortense watch my cats while I
am in the hospital?*

Then there are the recriminations of past choices: *Why
did I ever start smoking? Why can't I stop eating so much? I
should have gone to Europe when I had the chance. I should
have spent less time at work. I should have gone to the doctor
earlier.*

All of these mind trails are natural, despite knowing
that we cannot undo or change the past.

Give It All to God

This is, again, where God comes in. Giving everything to
God does not justify or right past choices and deeds, good
or bad. Giving everything to God, however, does allow God
to use the past for your future good. Past negative behaviors can be an impetus to help others avoid those behaviors,
once they are turned over to God. For example, regret for
smoking can help encourage a loved one to turn away from
smoking. A missed adventure, such as a trip to Europe, can
be channeled into encouraging someone else to go if they
have the chance — or it may become a high priority goal for
you to do as soon as you are able. By re-directing our regrets
into something positive, we can let them go and move on.
Channeling regrets into support for others, or action steps
for yourself, is freeing. By giving them to God, we open
ourselves to his transforming grace.

Go Deeper

Note that none of the questions most of us have in reviewing our lives really have much to do with medicine, at least in the short term. But they are related to lifestyle, duties, and responsibilities. You probably have an entire box of similar questions in your head right now. But there is another box of questions that go even deeper.

These more serious questions are applicable to everyone. But they are often buried. This is because no one really likes to ask these questions or deal with the answers: *Will I be alive next month? Next year? How did I get to this place? How did I get so far off track? Who loves me? Who will take care of me? Will I be okay? Will I be able to settle a longstanding difference or dispute before it's too late? Will anyone want to come to my funeral?*

These are fundamental and important questions.

Even if you are angry with God, you can take these questions to him. If you think he has totally abandoned you, you're wrong, but you certainly wouldn't be the first person to feel that way. Try to establish (or re-establish) your trust in him. Trust him, even if it is only for something tiny. The truth is that God has never stopped believing in you. The Book of Job in the Old Testament is full of the kinds of questions you might have, both from Job and from his friends and family. Consider reading the book, a synopsis of it, or find a podcast on Job and listen to it.

Open a Conversation About the Big Things

Only God knows the answer to some of the questions we have. Other questions we can pray about and then perhaps work on. Our own fears can be the biggest obstacles we face in trying to answer these questions, and many of us choose to set them aside instead of addressing them. Delaying a discussion of these topics just allows our own fears to grow. Honestly, those around us are wondering about the same things, so it reduces stress on all sides if you can just begin a dialogue.

Begin the conversation with God, and ask him to lead you to speaking with your loved ones. This is also another area where the caregiver may struggle more than the patient. Sometimes people are afraid that these discussions mean that the patient wants to give up or that the end is near. That may be true for some, but not for all. Even when there aren't many good answers, getting the questions out in the open is therapeutic. It allows all involved to start thinking about and looking for answers instead of being frozen in fear. Remember, God tells us, repeatedly, to not be afraid. So try opening the conversation and let fresh air and God's love touch those big questions we often prefer to ignore.

Some patients really do not want the answers to the bigger questions. If that is how you choose to handle it, that's up to you. If your doctor or caregiver brings up big questions, though, try to answer them. Your family and friends may need affirmations of love. Your medical team may need input that will help them do their best for you.

Build Relationships

Making contact with people can help you get back on the tracks. During the time I was in isolation, contact with others was very limited. On the few occasions someone stopped by with the Eucharist, I was almost always too sick to receive Holy Communion. So, due to the hassle of isolation procedures, they did not visit me often. I understood this, but it still felt like rejection — until one day, flipping through local television channels, I found my own parish priest offering Mass. I could not believe it. Our country house was next door to a small mission church. The priest, who lived in a small town about twenty miles away, came once a week for Sunday Mass. The odds of him being on a televised Mass, on a local channel in a big city over an hour away, had to be very slim. That day, I saw many of my parish friends and neighbors. Being in isolation at the time, this was a wonderful gift that I could not have even imagined. I knew that God had sent it to me as a surprise and to comfort me in my loneliness. So, if making friends or keeping up with them is not part of your skill set, especially when ill, do not worry. God is with you, and he will give you what you need when you need it, just as he did with me.

Be Inspired by the Apostles

If you are able, try reading the Acts of the Apostles in the Bible during this time. Written by Saint Luke, it is the story of the early Church. The first twelve chapters are mostly about Saint Peter, and then the story shifts more to Saint Paul, who would eventually write most of the New Testament letters. Considering that he was shipwrecked three times, beaten, stoned, lowered out of a window at night in a handmade basket, and thrown in jail a few times, what Paul accomplished is miraculous. Even more amazing is that Paul started out as one of the early Church's most powerful enemies. After realizing how off the track he was, in persecuting the early Christians, he got on the track toward God and never got off.

May we do the same.

Chapter Eight

IN THE PITS

But you, be self-possessed in all circumstances;
put up with hardship; perform the work
of an evangelist; fulfill your ministry.
— 2 TIMOTHY 4:5

There is no ignoring that hard times come to us all. When a major illness is involved, it is almost guaranteed. Treatments may fail, and the most basic capacities — or even body parts — may be lost. These things have happened to countless people since the beginning of time, but that does not help ease the burden when it is happening to you or someone you love. Three things can help us through these challenges: preparation, contemplative prayer, and a sense of humor.

1. Make Practical Preparations

As you learn more about your treatment or upcoming medical procedures, you may see patterns emerge in how you feel. For example, the first day or two after a treatment may be fine, but then, the third day, you can only lie in bed. Your symptoms may vary with extra stress or even with certain weather changes. You may learn you must budget your energy level so carefully that each activity must be planned and balanced against the energy needed for a future medical procedure or family event.

Do not worry about these issues. They are inevitable and, hopefully, passing. Even if they do linger, things will still get better as you learn how to manage your new situation. Being resentful will not help and only drags you down. Try, instead, to see it as a new game in which you can recognize new limitations but sneakily plan the things you most want to do anyway. Preparation is the key.

Set Priorities

No matter what your situation or stage in life, God comes first. Make connecting with him first thing in the morning a priority. Then look at how you can help someone else that day — say a prayer or find a way to be extra helpful to those you will see today. Then look at your situation. Resist making a laundry list of important things. Just focus on the most important.

Declutter

There are times when less is more, when simplicity is the goal. In the same way we clear out clutter and clean the house before a holiday, we should clear out the clutter and streamline our lives with a major illness. Decluttering brings a feeling of freedom. So, if you can physically do some of that, especially in the room where you will be resting, it is great. Some will not have the physical ability to actually move stuff around, make piles to donate, or put into storage. If that is the case, consider asking someone to help you.

Plan Ahead

Each condition or illness will have its own schedules and effects. But from a general perspective, there are some basic things to consider doing. On a spiritual level, every parish church I have attended has a list of people to pray for. Put yourself on it, whether that means asking a friend to do it for you or making the phone call yourself. There will also be a list for those wanting to receive the Holy Eucharist while homebound or in the hospital. If you are interested, ask if it is available.

On a more practical level, consider requesting, in advance, Meals on Wheels to be delivered to your home if bad times are on the horizon. (Often, a doctor's signature is required for this service.) Ask a friend to stock up a supply of your favorite comfort snacks and food. If you're able, fill the freezer with meals for future use.

Find out how to plan rides or taxis before you need them. At low times, even picking up the phone can be exhausting, so figure out as much as you can ahead of time.

Other things to plan are the weekly and daily things we usually do without thinking: grocery shopping, basic cleaning and cooking, and general shopping. Now is the time to splurge on things that may take some of the pressure off. It may be as simple as buying paper plates to cut down on dishes or hiring someone to clean once a week. If you have children, plan childcare for difficult days while you still feel good.

If you plan to keep working, make sure you have people in place to help you, even if you aren't sure you will ever need to ask them. Things such as arranging for rides to and from work, someone to deliver papers, or setting up dual monitors for your work computer at home can be vital.

Once you have the necessities in place, schedule at least one really nice positive thing. It can be as simple as setting out a favorite DVD, putting out a new birdfeeder that you can watch from the couch, or asking a friend to bring a favorite treat over on a Tuesday afternoon. If you are more ambitious, you can plan an activity such as a concert, movie, or manicure. Encourage your caregivers to do something nice for themselves as well. If you're having a bad day and are unable to enjoy something right then, that's okay and just part of the journey. Just save your planned treat for a better day and give yourself a pat on the back for planning it in the first place. Focus on the joy you received from the anticipation and just plan something else for next time.

Connect with Another's Struggle

Another way to prepare for harder times down the road is to read about or listen to others' struggles. Stories of people who have fought against the odds can be encouraging. Best-sellers sometimes document a survivor's struggles against nature or a difficult circumstance. There are also stories of saints and martyrs that might inspire you for the hard times ahead. And the Bible is full of stories of real people who had horrible things to contend with. Any of these choices can help you become closer to God by seeing how others have relied on God during harrowing times and survived. It is good to know that when we are at the bottom of the pit, God is with us. He still hears us. And we can always trust God to do what is best for us.

2. Prayer Without Words

The second thing that will help you when things are at their worst is a kind of prayer you may not have tried: contemplative prayer. As a child, I got the mistaken idea that contemplative prayer was only part of the lives of solitary monks and cloistered nuns. I'm not sure how I arrived at this, but I was wrong. Contemplative prayer is something we all can — and should — be open to, but especially in times of deep trouble. The *Catechism* quotes Saint Teresa of Ávila on the subject. Prayer, she wrote, "in my opinion is nothing else than a close sharing between friends; it means taking time frequently to be alone with him who we know loves us" (CCC 2709).

We should always make time for the Lord, but one of the gifts of a major illness is the quiet time we can spend with God. As future plans are disrupted and daily routines disturbed, time opens up. Personally, I learned that I could have been engaging in a lot more prayer of the contemplative kind all along rather than rote verbal prayers. I could have been building a deeper relationship with Jesus simply by spending time in his presence. I had ignored what I knew to be true, that

> One does not undertake contemplative prayer only when one has the time: one makes time for the Lord, with the firm determination not to give up, no matter what trials and dryness one may encounter. One cannot always meditate, but one can always enter into inner prayer, independently of the conditions of health, work, or emotional state. (CCC 2710)

This teaching speaks directly to those of us with major illnesses. Contemplative prayer is a way to visit with Jesus, no matter how sick or miserable we are, or how fragile our emotions.

Prayer without words is possible for everyone, but especially for those "in the pits" and also for their loving, but often exhausted, family members and caregivers. If possible, read, or have a caregiver read to you, the beautiful and inspiring section on contemplative prayer in the *Catechism*. It is only eleven paragraphs long (CCC 2709–2719), about two pages total. Even reading one paragraph per day could motivate you to begin the simple practice of being with God.

3. Keep a Sense of Humor

The third suggestion of how our faith can help anyone "in the pits" is with a sense of humor. Yes, the Catholic Church encourages us to have a sense of humor because God has a sense of humor. This humor is found easily in the stories of patron saints. Just as a saint's feast is usually tied to the date of their death, so their patronage is often tied to how they died. For example, Saint Lawrence, a deacon, was martyred during one of the Roman Empire's persecutions of the Church. He was burned to death on a large outside grill and allegedly told his torturers to turn him over because he was done on the first side. He is the patron saint of grill cooks.

I have gone through various stages with this type of story. As a child, I thought it tragic. And it is. Later, I thought it was funny, but a rather cruel joke on poor Saint Lawrence! Now I understand that the Church is claiming this atrocity and holding it close to her heart on our behalf. It is a bold declaration of, yes, this happened to one of us, and the powers of evil thought they had won. But we know better, because Saint Lawrence is now in heaven and that means we have the last laugh, as it were. This is the kind of laughter in the face of death we can claim as our spiritual heritage.

In any case, add funny movies and plays to your list of entertainment for the days when you need to rest.

Claim Your Cross

In chapter 12 of his Gospel, Saint Luke wrote that Jesus told his followers not to fear those who kill the body. Now, medical personnel are obviously not trying to kill us, but it may seem close to that when the conversation includes things like removing a foot, leg, or breast. Sometimes it takes time to slow down our emotions upon hearing such news, to let the rational, reasoning mind take over. It is not easy, but it is possible. We, too, can claim our cross as our own and take it up as Jesus did, as Saint Lawrence did.

Emulating a Catholic sense of humor can be especially helpful for those who through illness or treatment lose part of their body. There's no getting around the fact that this is traumatic. Even if the alternative is death, and we know that it must be done to survive, it is still traumatic. As with any trauma, there is shock, as well as sadness, doubt, and the psychological issues of actually, physically losing part of yourself. Questions of how you'll need to adapt and what your future life will be like arise. Sometimes the questions include things that have nothing to do with medicine: *Will I still be loved? Will I ever be attractive again? Will I be able to return to my old job?* These are all valid questions, but it is doubtful that satisfactory answers will be immediately forthcoming. Breathe deeply and try to keep the emotions under control without squelching them. In other words, express what you feel to someone you trust, and then do your best to move on.

Quite often, patients do not really have much of a choice. But that is an opportunity to learn how to humbly accept the realities we face and embrace them as much as possible. Accepting this cross, trying to carry it gently and with Jesus beside you, will not only get you through it but will also give you something good as well. Uniting your pain and loss to the pain and loss that Jesus experienced will give you strength and fortitude. This, in turn, will lighten the burden of the doctors and nurses, and also that of your friends and relatives who are suffering along with you — even though you may not think so. Sometimes we think that our burdens don't count as crosses, or that we have to choose our own sacrifices in order for them to count. This is not true, and we need only to look at the saints to prove it.

Pick a Patron

You may not be familiar with many saints. Almost everyone in North America, Catholic or not, could name the Virgin Mary, Joseph, and Francis of Assisi. The next rung would probably add in John the Baptist, some biblical characters like Moses and David, and the four Gospel writers: Matthew, Mark, Luke, and John. Catholics would know some saints from any churches they have attended, from family names, and maybe from some recently canonized saints such as Mother Teresa of Kolkata and Pope John Paul II. For most of us, beyond that it gets pretty murky. After all, it is two thousand years of history, and it's not as if everyone is talking about saints on a regular basis!

At this time in your life, it's probably best to forget the image of someone who was pious from childhood and spent all day praying. There are saints like that. But for right now, it's probably better to find someone who suffered, maybe even in a way similar to what you are suffering. As a woman who required a mastectomy due to breast cancer, I discovered Saint Agatha. Her breasts were cut off as part of the torture she endured before her martyrdom in the year 251. Her circumstances and mine were completely different, but we had the loss of a body part in common. I truly felt better praying with someone who had at least some of the same fears and pain and questions that I had, even if it was centuries ago. Today, Saint Agatha is still part of our family's prayers, and I try to make it to Mass on her feast day to thank her for her help.

Consider looking for a patron saint, one that understands your loss but who can keep reminding you to look at the bigger picture of salvation and redemption. Find someone who will help you develop that sense of joy — and, yes, humor — that can overcome any loss. Finding the right saint doesn't take long. Just ask the Lord to show you.

It was important to me to find a saint who had similar physical issues as mine. On the other hand, you may not want to be reminded of your recent problems, and that is okay. But still look for a saint who can be beside you during this journey. If nothing else, it helps to be learning new things that are not medical in nature.

To get you started, here is a list of some saints that may apply to those with serious medical issues. For starters there is Saint Peregrine, the patron saint for those with cancer. He is usually pictured holding up a black tunic so that one can see the cancer on his leg. Saint Dymphna helps those with mental health issues. Saint John of God is invoked for heart ailments. Saint Lucy is well known for helping those with afflictions of the eye. Saint Josemaría Escrivá and Saint Paulina of Brazil both suffered from diabetes. Consider adding prayers to Saint Luke and the recent Saints Gianna Beretta Molla and Guiseppe Moscati, who were physicians, for your own doctors. There are also saints for nurses such as Saint Irene, who tended Saint Sebastian, or read about the Wild West's Sister Blandina Segale, who nursed a member of Billy the Kid's gang back to health.

Choose Media Carefully

While reading saint stories can help strengthen your faith, put your concerns into perspective, and increase your love for the Church, just be sure it helps you remain positive. It helped me to read about the saints, but it may not help you. If the story you pick up is gruesome or depressing to you, put it down and look for something else.

This can happen with other forms of media as well. A friend gave me a "great" movie, totally forgetting that in the first fifteen minutes of the film, the mom dies of the same cancer I had. I was upset, but I knew she must have forgotten that part. Sure enough, when I next spoke with her, she admitted that she didn't remember that part until a week later, and then she was afraid to call me. We were able to laugh about it and move on.

Use the Tools You Have

If at all possible, prepare yourself for any hard times ahead by receiving the sacraments in advance. If needed, ask for help in finding televised Masses and in scheduling a time to receive the Sacrament of Reconciliation and Holy Communion. Begin practicing contemplative prayer by purposefully choosing to spend time with God in silence. Let the saints lighten your heart, and re-affirm your faith with their stories. The inevitable times of being "in the pits" will not magically disappear, but they will feel shorter — and they can produce light, not only for yourself but for those around you. And that is a beautiful thing.

Chapter Nine

A "NEW NORMAL"

Seek out the LORD and his might;
constantly seek his face.
— PSALM 105:4

Whenever good news comes and whatever it is, celebrate it. Perhaps a change in medication means that you'll be able to avoid bad side effects. Maybe your treatment worked better than expected and you can end it earlier. Maybe you get permission to leave the hospital. Or maybe your "numbers" are better than they were. The celebration may be lower-key than what you are used to, but that is okay. Be sure to tell everyone who has been concerned for you when there's something to celebrate, and thank them for their prayers.

Say "Thank You"

Remember to thank your nurses and doctors as well. Recently, my daughter, who is a nurse, came home from a twelve-hour shift very happy that one of her favorite patients had received some good news. After several days in the cardiovascular ICU, this gentleman's only request was that one of the nurses take a picture of him when he could finally sit up so that he could send it to his family. It turned out he was everyone's favorite patient. Why? Because, my daughter explained, "he is always so grateful and thankful for anything we do. And believe me, that never happens."

I hope that was an exaggeration after a long night, but grateful patients are rare. So celebrate with the staff of the clinic or hospital as well when you get good news.

Be Flexible

After celebrating good news, there may well be new challenges, but do not fear. Remember Saint Paul's words in Philippians 4:13: "I have the strength for everything through him who empowers me." It may take some help — again — and a new shifting of schedules — again. But there is always a way to receive whatever is happening as a gift. You are still alive and becoming closer to God, hour by hour, day by day.

If you have been hospitalized, a different schedule of medications may be necessary when you are released to return home. It may seem like a hassle, but remember that going home *is* still something to celebrate. Others can help with paper schedules or setting alarms on your phone, whatever it takes to get new medications and treatments straightened out so that the new routine runs smoothly.

I hope it is not the case for you, but sometimes people do not feel that certain medical personnel are listening to them. You may find that calling the nurse or pharmacist, instead of the doctor, is more productive. Dealing with the medical world can sap your energy when you are already low. If you don't already do so, now is the time to take a relative or close friend to appointments with you as a support and patient advocate.

Transportation may be more of a challenge after leaving the hospital. There will almost certainly be various medical visits for follow up. If transport might be a problem, talk to the nurse or social worker at the hospital before you leave. There are volunteers and public vans that can help if you need it, or if you prefer not to burden relatives or friends.

New Fears

For some, clinic visits and hospital stays can provide a sense of security. But it's easy to dislike the hospital atmosphere, with its regimented routines and interruptions. That's why the desire to get back home is huge for many of us. At the beginning of a major illness, it is difficult to give up your independence. But upon returning home and regaining some autonomy, renewed independence may lead to new fears: *Will I remember my medication? My appointments? What if I get sick again? What if something goes wrong?*

Regaining independence is a good goal; it is also an adjustment. In a hospital, someone is always around to help. That's probably not the case once you go home. First of all, remind yourself to relax, because the staff would not have released you unless they were confident you could proceed on your own. Second, it is possible to prepare for these rational fears to a certain extent. For example, train yourself to always keep a cell phone with you. If need be, ask a friend if they could find you a jacket or sweatshirt with zippered pockets so that you always have your phone at hand. In some circumstances, county health services can call you at a prearranged time each day to check in and see how you are doing.

Do not be disappointed in yourself for having these concerns. It shows you are thoughtful and intelligent, that you realize there are still challenges ahead. You have made it this far, so you should know that, with God beside you, you can handle anything!

Managing Medications

In the hospital, someone brought your medication at the right time and made sure you took it. Now *you* are responsible for those medications. If there are numerous medications involved, there needs to be a plan of how to take them. That can become even more complicated if some can go together and some can't; if some must be taken with food and others on an empty stomach; some two hours from bedtime, and so on. Do not be afraid to ask for help to make a medication schedule. The local pharmacy can be a good place to start. It's convenient to ask when you or your caregiver picks up the medications.

It's important to be aware that medications may need to be adjusted. In fact, they may need to be adjusted several times. If you are struggling with negative side effects, contact your doctor sooner rather than later. This is not being a "problem patient." It is being a proactive, intelligent patient, who wants to manage his or her health as much as possible. Ask if there are alternatives that you can try if something isn't working well for you. This may be a long and frustrating process. Often, there is really not much you can do about it except to keep charts of reactions, sensitivities, times taken, and food ingested.

You are not a poor helpless patient. Picture yourself instead as an architect who must go over and over the same plans until they are right for the job. Or as an actor who has to repeat the same scene over and over until the director is satisfied. It may even help to see your medications as a puzzle or mystery to be solved — because it really is!

A Dose of Prayer

After making a schedule, double-check it. Once the prescription schedule is set, consider adding a very short prayer to each pill time slot. For example, if you have a prescription that is taken three times a day, you could pair it with praying the Angelus, which is normally prayed three times a day. If that seems too daunting, make up your own prayer or say a short prayer like the short Divine Mercy prayer, "Jesus, I trust in you." If you have medications which must be refrigerated, ask a friend for a magnet or two, with a prayer or Bible verse, to stick on the refrigerator door when it is time to take those meds. Do not make praying at these times an extra burden. Keep it short — just seconds even.

When you have adjusted to being home and are in your new normal schedule, do not forget to keep in contact with God. It is hard to keep a friendship going when you never visit, so make time for God on a daily basis. In fact, try to schedule time throughout the day, just to check in. There are many ways to do this, and you can choose whatever and whenever works best for you.

A basic plan could be saying "Good morning" to Jesus before you get out of bed and then making a morning offering, telling God that you give the day to him and will be on the lookout for his grace and blessings. Prayers at every meal in thanksgiving, not only for the food but also for your life, is an easy habit to start. Add a simple night prayer and you have six short connections throughout the day. You could add in the Angelus at 6 a.m., noon, and 6 p.m., as well as a visit with Jesus during a short review of the day before sleep. The purpose of a review is to notice how God was present to you during the day. It also helps to identify the opportunities for grace and mercy you took advantage of as well as those you missed. If your strength increases, consider finding a televised Mass to watch on television or to listen to on the radio.

The benefits of daily Mass are wonderful, if you can manage the hardest part and just get yourself there. Of course, there may be no possible way for you to get there, and it is unwise to even try unless you are at a point where you can travel and have the energy to be out and about. But once you feel up to it, see if you can fit at least one weekday Mass within your week, in addition to Sunday. Attending those quiet, uncrowded Masses can give you peace and help you to set the priorities for your day and your life. I found that no matter how little time I had in my day, chores and errands and events — even naps — always seemed to go more smoothly if I was able to make Mass part of my morning.

Ask God to lead you — not only to a new, but an even better "normal."

Chapter Ten

THE JOURNEY HOME

*Whom else have I in the heavens? / None beside
you delights me on earth. / Though my flesh and my heart
fail, / God is the rock of my heart, my portion forever.*
— PSALM 73:25–26

For some, this major illness will be the vehicle that takes you out of this world and into the next. The journey through death is frightening to think about, and even more daunting to make. Yet, we all must travel it eventually.

Death is usually seen as something we should fight. This is true in a sense. Our faith teaches that we should do our best to keep healthy so that we can continue God's work here on earth. But there are times we learn that death is on our horizon sooner than we had planned. When that happens, we can come to a place where we can trust that God's plan is best. That, however, isn't easy.

Let God Be God

Once when visiting with my dad, who was 97 at the time, we found ourselves discussing the day's obituaries. "Who wants to live to be one hundred anyway? Nobody!" he commented. Then he paused and added, "Unless you are ninety-nine." There is so much truth in that!

God must sometimes shake his head in wonder at us. We all know we'll die someday, but the tendency is to avoid thinking about it. That is why a major illness can be a real grace. Confronting a serious diagnosis forces us to recognize that death is a reality we may no longer be able to ignore, and that it can come sooner rather than later. Hopefully, that realization turns hearts toward our eternal home and helps us continue that focus for the remainder of the time we have. It should also inspire us to help those we will be leaving behind by settling the legal, funereal, and financial issues they will otherwise face.

Settle What You Can

Legal and financial issues, in the great scheme of things, are of little importance to you if you are dying. If you ever thought you could take it with you, it should be obvious by now that you cannot. However, straightening out your temporal affairs is a great blessing to those who live on after you. Even simple things can be very helpful.

Putting a designated name with a TOD (transfer on death) on the back of your car title will save endless headaches for someone. Ask someone to check any life insurance policies you may have, and make sure a beneficiary is listed on each one. Ask a relative or coworker to help you check any relevant policies in place, and determine if anything needs to be signed. If you own a house, confirm that it will go to the person you want to have it. If you have put off making a will, do not panic. Just have your closest caretaker call a local attorney and ask if he or she will either come to see you or take your instructions over the phone and come to the hospital or hospice for a signature. Thinking of others as much as you are able and doing what you can to make sure your loved ones are not thrown into a huge mess upon your death are good things. Take these steps as soon as possible so that you can keep your focus on God, not the things you are preparing to leave behind.

Care for Your Soul

Spiritual needs should be at the top of our list at every point in our lives. We all know that this often does not happen. But as we approach the end of this life, caring for our souls ought to take prime position. There is nothing more important than getting right with God, and others. For Catholics, that means receiving the Sacrament of Reconciliation and the Sacrament of the Sick. These are the single most important things you can do as you approach your journey home. Do not wait. If things turn around and good health returns, you may receive these sacraments again (CCC 1515). If you are a caregiver and your loved one is not alert, call a priest anyway. A person does not have to be conscious to receive grace.

The logistics of this are simple, and there are various options. The first is for you or your caregiver to simply call your parish priest. This is appropriate whether you are at home, at a rehab facility, in hospice, or in the hospital. If you are in the hospital, ask the nurse to contact the Catholic chaplain for you. Sometimes the chaplain is a lay person. Don't worry! When you need a priest, that person will find one for you. Other hospital chaplains may not be Catholic, but they will still be helpful. If they offer a blessing in the meantime, by all means feel free to accept it. Remember that you can — and should — always request a Catholic priest.

Our first daughter was born prematurely. No first-time parent plans to have a three-pound, sick baby, and both my husband and I were in shock. She was fine, at first, for a baby that size, but took a sudden turn for the worse. As we watched from the doorway, we saw one doctor, then another, and then more and more nurses crowd around her open bassinet. We were not allowed to enter, as there was barely enough room for the medical staff. When a nurse came to us crying, we knew it was really, really bad.

We asked the nurse to call for a priest, and she immediately did so. We were at a large, secular university hospital and worried that our daughter would not make it until a priest could come. But a priest lived somewhere on campus and answered the phone — while in the shower! He did not even finish his shower, but just threw on his clothes and ran to the neonatal ICU. The medical staff was still desperately working on our baby, but they made way for the wet-haired priest to baptize her. Afterward, he came over and told us she wasn't nearly as blue as some preemies he had seen. This sounds funny now, but it was music to our ears then. He stayed with us until they had her stabilized. This was a great grace for our daughter, and for us.

According to the *Catechism of the Catholic Church* (1499–1532), the Sacrament of the Sick benefits us in four ways. First, it is a *"particular grace of the Holy Spirit,"* which gives strength, peace, and courage to cope with illness or old age, and it helps a person to resist "discouragement and anguish in the face of death" (CCC 1520, emphasis in original). Second, it helps a sick person to unite his own suffering to that of Christ (CCC 1521). Third, in a spiritual exchange, the sacrament enables the Church to help you, but it also empowers you to help the Church and all those who suffer (CCC 1522). Last, it is a *"preparation for the final journey"* (CCC 1523, emphasis in original). Those who must lovingly accompany their loved ones as they journey toward death may also find some solace in the Church's confidence in how God works in our lives — even up to the last second.

Call on Saint Joseph

Also remember throughout this time that Saint Joseph, the foster father of Jesus and spouse of the Virgin Mary, is the patron of a "happy death." Saint Joseph is a true wonder-worker. As the man who cared for Mary and Jesus, Joseph understands the difficulties of family life. Concerns about family are often paramount at this time, so don't hesitate to ask Saint Joseph to help your family. Depending on your circumstances as a patient, ask his help for the energy and strength to make the plans for your family that are still left to be done. As a caregiver, consider asking for strength and peace for both yourself and your loved ones.

Love in Advance

There are things you can do to ensure that your family and friends know just how much you love them. Think ahead and consider prearranging or asking a friend to send flowers on special days or occasions in the next year to your spouse or a son or daughter whose graduation or wedding you may miss. Another thing to think about is contacting your parish office to have Masses offered for you and your family after your death. The stipend for these Masses is small, and they can be scheduled in advance, maybe even for special days such as a wedding anniversary or birthday or the anniversary of your death. This request can also be included in your will.

Make Funeral Arrangements

Everyone knows it is best to have funeral arrangements figured out in advance, but if you haven't done that yet, just do it now. Funeral home representatives will usually come to wherever you are to help you consider your options and make plans. It is so much easier on those you love to do this together and in advance.

None of us wants this task on our to-do list. We don't want to think about it, even when we know we are dying. But if you can handle even part of the planning, doing so will lift the burden off those you love.

Make an appointment to discuss your plans for the funeral with the parish staff, if you are able, or ask a family member, friend, or caretaker to do it on your behalf. Though the rite itself is set, and beautiful, you are usually able to choose the Scripture readings and music. There are also choices to be made about how people will pay their respects, as well as how your bodily remains will be laid to rest. Both traditional burial and cremation are permitted by the Church. Remember to ask Saint Joseph to help you.

Be Open to Grace

Opening yourself to God's graces is the most important thing you can do when death is near. If you avail yourself of the sacraments, you will begin to look forward to meeting Jesus face-to-face. That will bring you peace. This is a time to pray without ceasing in any and every way possible. By doing so, you will not only find comfort yourself, but affect the people closest to you, as well as those you will never see or know. Your example will speak volumes to those you love, to the staff, and to strangers walking down the hall who notice a priest coming to your room or hear hymns softly sung by friends and family members. To be a witness to your faith, even to the last breath, would be a most beautiful offering to others — and most importantly, to the Lord you have grown close to through this experience.

Chapter Eleven

A Pilgrimage of Joy and Thanksgiving

*Rejoice in the Lord always. I shall say it again:
rejoice! Your kindness should be known to all.
The Lord is near. Have no anxiety at all, but
in everything, by prayer and petition, with
thanksgiving, make your requests known to
God. Then the peace of God that surpasses
all understanding will guard your hearts
and minds in Christ Jesus.*
— Philippians 4:4–7

Whether your medical journey is short and intense, a chronic condition you must continue to live with, or a terminal illness, your serious diagnosis has the potential to bring you closer to God. Although illness is not something anyone would choose, the challenge you are facing — or helping your friend or family member to face — can actually help you find joy, thankfulness, and redemption. Strange as it may seem, you can become the best person you have ever been, even when you are feeling your absolute worst. That happens when we learn how to place not only our circumstances, but ourselves, into God's hands.

Take a Vacation with God

After asking you so many times to not focus on yourself, I would like you to plan one thing for yourself — a pilgrimage. A pilgrimage is a trip of thanksgiving and joy for whatever graces you have received. For some, it will be thankfulness for healing. For others, it will be a thankfulness for God's presence and prayers for that continued presence while waiting for death. Take some time and plan a pilgrimage that fills your heart with joy. If for some reason it falls through, remember that God will use even the planning to give you the grace you need! He loves you so much and knows the desires of your heart. He sees that your pilgrimage — wherever it takes you — is a way for you to find him, to praise him, and to grow closer to him.

A pilgrimage by its very nature focuses our attention on God, while also doing something that helps us look at the whole of our lives. Serious illness is full of different kinds of challenges and lessons. There is much to absorb and learn on so many different levels that it can be overwhelming. So, when the end of this particular journey is near, whether that be a new normal of continued lifetime treatment, a return to health, or a chance to prepare for death, plan a pilgrimage. Go as big as you can, given your circumstances. Some may be able to go to the Holy Land, Rome, or a place linked to a favorite saint. Most, though, are more likely to drive to a nearby shrine or stay at a special place for a night or two.

There is no set schedule — just plan your own. Allow time, though, for silent prayer and thanksgiving for all those wonderful gifts written in your gratitude journal, including the things you were too sick to note at the time. Find the schedule for confession and attend when it is available. It is humbling to consider that we can sin in thoughts and words even when we are not as physically capable as we usually are! Yet the renewal that confession gives surpasses any regret or guilt that has built up along with bad behaviors or habits.

Keep the Gifts You Have Received

A pilgrimage also provides the time and space to reflect on what you have been through. Maybe your illness has provided time to already do this — perhaps many times — but this time can be a deeper reflection of how your relationship with God has changed. It can also be a time for you to strategize about how to keep hold of what you have gained. Are you better at seeing the good in your life and thanking God for it? Do you trust him more than ever before? How have you grown closer to God? Have you grown closer to any particular saint? How has the way you pray changed?

Do not rush a pilgrimage once you have begun it. Leave free time for God to speak to your heart, and to give you rest. Thank him for all the graces you have received and continue to receive. Ask him to let you feel his presence. It doesn't *have* to be a religious place, but consider finding one, especially if that is not something you have done before.

Embrace Simplicity

Oftentimes, energy and finances have taken a huge hit over the course of illness. If so, ask around for a local shrine, retreat center, monastery, or convent. There are also cathedrals and basilicas we can visit. It is surprising how many small shrines are scattered throughout the world. With the internet, it is easy to find Catholic sites throughout North America and beyond.

A pilgrimage need not be elaborate. In fact, the simpler it is, the better it may be. It is just a time to pray and reflect, a chance to receive the sacraments of Reconciliation and Holy Eucharist — if possible, all in a special place. A pilgrimage is a perfect way to thank God for his help and to ask his continuing help in whatever happens next.

For some, a pilgrimage might represent the end of your medical challenge. For others, it will be a last hurrah before transitioning to new life in eternity with the Lord. In either case, a pilgrimage will provide you a chance to look back and see how God gave you the grace to endure difficult times, how hope sustained you, and how you have experienced that God was — and is — always by your side.

For all, I hope it is a time for looking forward to what is next, knowing that everything you have given to God remains always in his loving hands.